YOUR KNOWLEDGE HAS VALUE

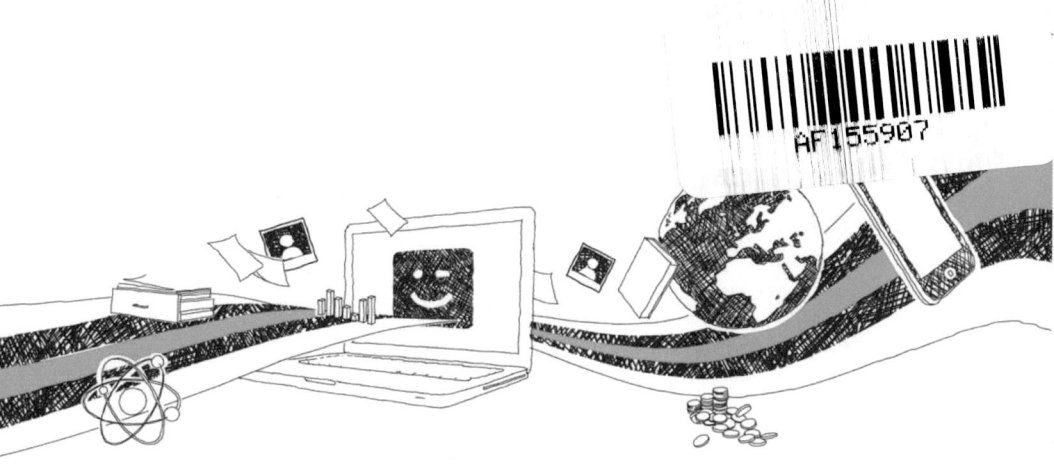

- We will publish your bachelor's and
  master's thesis, essays and papers

- Your own eBook and book -
  sold worldwide in all relevant shops

- Earn money with each sale

Upload your text at www.GRIN.com
and publish for free

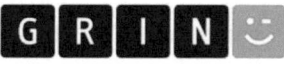

Bibliographic information published by the German National Library:

The German National Library lists this publication in the National Bibliography;
detailed bibliographic data are available on the Internet at http://dnb.dnb.de .

Imprint:

Copyright © 2006 GRIN Verlag, Open Publishing GmbH
Print and binding: Books on Demand GmbH, Norderstedt Germany
ISBN: 9783668368743

This book at GRIN:

http://www.grin.com/en/e-book/110867/the-cult-of-citizenship-education-by-a-
sears-and-e-hyslop-margison-a

Michael Ernest Sweet

The Cult of Citizenship Education by A. Sears and E. Hyslop-Margison. A Review

GRIN Publishing

GRIN - Your knowledge has value

Since its foundation in 1998, GRIN has specialized in publishing academic texts by students, college teachers and other academics as e-book and printed book. The website www.grin.com is an ideal platform for presenting term papers, final papers, scientific essays, dissertations and specialist books.

Visit us on the internet:

http://www.grin.com/

http://www.facebook.com/grincom

http://www.twitter.com/grin_com

The Cult of Citizenship Education

Reviewed by Michael Ernest Sweet

Concordia University Montreal

September 18, 2006

The Cult of Citizenship Education

"A dread that goes beyond the breakdown of bowling leagues and civic clubs… the fear of our young as letterless, unassailable barbarians"

(Pinsky, 2002).

Alan Sears and Emery Hyslop-Margison, in *The Cult of Citizenship Education*, illuminate the driving discourse behind the seeming explosion in democratic citizenship education reform with particular attention to the last decade.

Sears and Hyslop-Margison lay a solid foundation of scholarship to support their claim of a climate of educational reform driven by mere slogans and dogma, rather than any meaningful research or reliable data. Calling on Janice Gross Stein's 2001 Massey Lectures, *The Cult of Efficiency*, Sears and Hyslop-Margison, in accessible terms, explain that meaningful dialogue around issues of educational reform is precluded by the participants being caught up in a maze of rapid-fire rhetoric. As a result, *The Cult of Citizenship Education*, is a call for a more careful, thoughtful, and nuanced approach in understanding and promoting democratic citizenship education and its reform.

Moving forward, Sears and Hyslop-Margison begin to analyze some of the rhetoric produced by this cult mentality. Their overarching claim is that a grossly distorted discourse of crisis has formed around the subject of citizenship education, and is a driving force in sweeping reforms resulting in little to no value in regards to meaningful reform. Sears and Hyslop-Margison synthesize the discourse of crisis into three main areas (1) the crisis of ignorance, (2) the crisis of alienation, and (3) the crisis of agnosticism. Calling forward a host of reputable scholars and research they attempt to disassemble these claims. Without wishing to compromise the integrity of their arguments, I will further summarize them for our purposes here.

Within the crisis of ignorance Sears and Hyslop-Margison assert that our youth are no more ignorant than that of a hundred years ago, and that which they are ignorant of is

YOUR KNOWLEDGE HAS VALUE

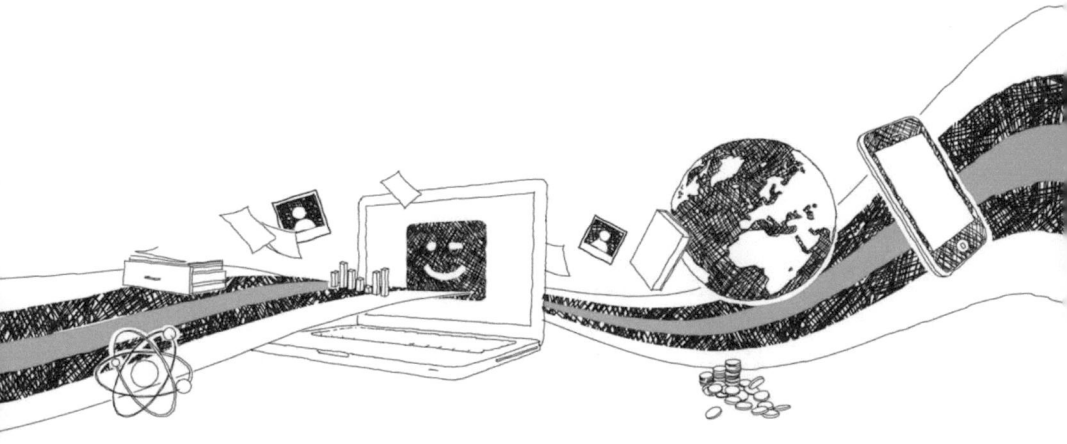

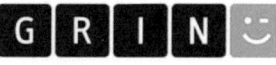

Gavin Hutchison

Drugs and Drug Use. Understandings of the Term 'Addiction'

GRIN Publishing

Bibliographic information published by the German National Library:

The German National Library lists this publication in the National Bibliography; detailed bibliographic data are available on the Internet at http://dnb.dnb.de .

Imprint:

Copyright © 2015 GRIN Verlag, Open Publishing GmbH
Print and binding: Books on Demand GmbH, Norderstedt Germany
ISBN: 978-3-668-01064-2

This book at GRIN:

http://www.grin.com/en/e-book/288683/drugs-and-drug-use-understandings-of-the-term-addiction

GRIN - Your knowledge has value

Since its foundation in 1998, GRIN has specialized in publishing academic texts by students, college teachers and other academics as e-book and printed book. The website www.grin.com is an ideal platform for presenting term papers, final papers, scientific essays, dissertations and specialist books.

Visit us on the internet:

http://www.grin.com/

http://www.facebook.com/grincom

http://www.twitter.com/grin_com

<u>Different understandings of 'addiction' exist and have existed at different times. Discuss such</u>
<u>understandings and their strengths and weaknesses.</u>

In contemporary discourse 'addiction' can be applied to any number of behaviours or activities. For example "[i]n today's society, we have sex-aholics, choc-aholics, work-aholics, shop-aholics, and golf-aholics. We have self-help programs called overeaters-anonymous, gamblersanonymous, internet-sex-anonymous, and smokers-anonymous." (Boyd, J. 1999) This recent discourse of addiction can be manipulated by 'addicts' to justify their behaviour, and to create sympathy towards them. Those claiming addiction may in fact not be an addict, however they now realise it is now more socially acceptable to be deemed an 'addict' than just participant in 'addictive' behaviors. This essay will concern itself with discourses of addiction to drugs. Understandings of addiction to substances such as narcotics, tobacco and alcohol have been conceptualised and re conceptualised throughout recent history. Early biological and pharmacological theories of addiction still dictate policy on 'addictive' substances, however social and psychological theories have gained momentum and explain aspects of addiction biological theories do not.

It is important to gain an insight into attitudes towards the concept of addiction before substances were conceptualised as being addictive. "Prior to the 19th century, the English word "addiction" had a traditional meaning...To be "addicted", meant either to be legally given over to somebody as a bond-slave, or, more broadly, to have given oneself over, or devoted oneself, to somebody or something." (Alexander, B. N.D) Addiction had nothing to do with substances, this however changed.

The work of Levine, H. (1978) gives an insight into American attitudes before alcohol was conceptualised as an addictive substance. He claims that "[d]uring the colonial period most people were not concerned with drunkenness; it was neither especially troublesome nor stigmatized behavior..." However many powerful colonials began to complain about the amount of drunkenness, and "[b]y the 1760s... Benjamin Franklin labeled taverns "a Pest to Society."" (Levine, H. 1978) People who were found to be drunk on a regular occasion became stigmatised, "they called such people drunkards...Occasionally they described drunkards as addicted to drunkenness or intemperance... In the colonial period "addicted" meant habituated, and one was habituated to drunkenness, not to liquor." (Levine, H. 1978) This distinction is important, as it can be seen that it is not the substances that were seen as addictive, it is the behavior attached to the consumption that is. "In the traditional view...the drunkard's sin was the love of "excess" drink to the point of drunkenness." (Levine, H. 1978) Addictive behavior toward the consumption of alcohol was viewed as a choice. "Drunkenness was a choice, albeit a sinful one, which some individuals made." (Levine, H. 1978) This understanding views addiction as a habit. This theory is problematic. 'Love' is seen as the reason for drunkenness, however psychological reasons may

1

have affected the desire to drink. Also those who may feel as though their indulgence was a problem were not offered any help, instead they were seen as criminals, "[t]owns circulated lists of common drunkards, and landlords who sold liquor to them could be fined or have their licenses revoked. Some drunkards were punished severely." (Levine, H. 1978) However addiction was seen as a choice, which is contrary to the later disease model.

The work of Dr. Rush. B (cited in Levine, H. 1978) could be described as the foundations for contemporary understandings of the disease model of addiction. "Rush organized the developing medical and commonsense wisdom into a distinctly new paradigm. According to Rush, drunkards were "addicted" to spirituous liquors; and they became addicted gradually and progressively..." (Levine, H. 1978) The shift from addiction to being drunk to addiction to the substance laid the foundations for medical theories of addiction. It also implied the pharmacological structure of the substance affected the possibility of becoming addicted. Rushs work has many similarities to modern discourses of addiction, for example "he clearly described the drunkard's condition as loss of control over drinking behavior – as compulsive activity; third, he declared the condition to be a disease; and fourth, he prescribed total abstinence as the only way to cure the drunkard..." The use of the medical term disease changed those seen as addicts from criminals into people who needed specialised medical help. These principles where adopted by the temperance movement and later by Alcoholics Anonymous, both went on to argue that "persons... have lost control over their drinking". (Levine, H. 1978) The temperance movement shifted it's focus from addiction to prohibition, and thus the disease model lost its popularity. "The drunkard came to be viewed less and less as a victim, and more and more as simply a pest and menace." (Levine, H. 1978)

The disease concept of addiction re-emerged through alcoholics anonymous during the 1930s and 1940s. Its re-emergence was the catalyst for a new medical discourse of addiction. Hyman, S. et al, (2001:695) claims that "[a]ddiction can appropriately be considered as a chronic medical illness." The brains reaction to addictive substances has been widely explored. Research into a "brain neurochemical called dopamine has revived interest in the possibility that a common brain mechanism may be involved in pleasure and reward." (Gossop, M. 2007:29) "'[t]he mesolimbic dopamine system... provides pleasure in the process of rewarding certain behavior' (Blum et al. 1996 cited in Lende, D et al, 2001:448) Gossop, M. (2007:29) assesses research which shows dopamine is linked to "the 'wanting' component of motivation." Hyman, S. et al, (2001: 696) explains "[a]ddictive drugs are both rewarding (interpreted by the brain as intrinsically positive) and reinforcing (behaviours associated with such drugs tend to be repeated)" Reward and reinforcement of drug effects lead the brain to want more. Gossops, M. (2007:29) explains this is because "a number of changes occur in the brain that make the reward system hypersensitive (sensitized) to the effects of drugs. The sensitized brain appears to play a central role in determining those aspects of reward that lead to the experiences of 'wanting' and 'needing'." These "[m]olecular changes in the brain promote continued drug taking that becomes increasingly difficult for the individual to control." (Hyman, S. et al, 2001:696) This "powerful control over behaviour exerted by addictive drugs is thought to result from the brain's inability to distinguish between the activation of reward circuitry by naturally rewarding activities, such as eating, and the consumption of drugs" (Hyman, S. et al 2001:697)

However, if addiction were based on the premise of pleasure and reward one would assume that during the first experience the 'user' would feel "unambiguous pleasure." (Gossop, M.2007:27) This is often not the case, Gossip, M. (2007:27) states that "many people find their first experience...distinctly unpleasant: only later do they enjoy the effects." This raises the question, why do people continue to use? Also by using the term 'needing' this model suggests that users will find it extremely difficult to just stop using, as we will find out this is not always the case. The disease model also seems to assume all 'addicts' will respond the same to an addiction. Using drugs as an example we can confidently say "[t]he drug addict is not an evil, vicious and deprived monster, nor is he or she a perfectly normal person suffering from a metabolic disease. Addicts are individuals." (Gossop, M. 2007:191) Not all users will become addicts, and not all addicts lose control over their 'needs.' Some people who are seen to have an addiction still have their free will. I suggest that sometimes an addiction is an escape route from unbearable situations. Use is often less or stopped once that situation is elevated. Using the Vietnam War as a case study we can see that this can happen.

The Vietnam War and drug use amongst the American armed forces is key to this assertion. "As many as 20 per cent of the troops reported that they had been addicted to opiates... After discharge from the army only 7 per cent used any opiate drug, and only 1 per cent felt they had been addicted to drugs since their return" (Gossop, M. 2007:31) If these statistics are taken at face value, then the statement "[m]olecular changes in the brain promote continued drug taking that becomes increasingly difficult for the individual to control.." (Hyman, S. et al, 2001:696) is flawed. However these statistics are subject to scrutiny, at the very least how do we know these soldiers are being truthful? Working on the assumption they are truth, it is clear that a different understanding of addiction needs to be assessed.

Social or environmental experiences and situation give us a different understanding of addiction. Gossop, M. (2007:32-33) writes "[t]he young men who served in Vietnam were removed from their normal social environment and from many of its usual social and moral restraints...As a form of inward desertion, drugs represented a way of altering the nature of subjective reality itself, and for the US servicemen drugs were cheap and freely available." There are many social and environmental issues which combine to aid the process to addiction. "Psychologically, the experience of suddenly being removed from a safe, familiar environment to a strange, foreign and extremely threatening one increases pressure on the individual to take drugs." (Gossop, M. 2007:33) Gossop, M. (2007:33) also writes that drugs are a useful means of coping with fear, boredom and the physical strains of war. He also explains that peer pressure and availability were also factors towards the development of an addiction. This understanding of addiction is useful as it can be applied to many different settings. We can see why people start to become addicts, and not just what happens inside their bodies. It can be argued that a change of social setting and the removal of moral restraints gives us and a different understanding of addiction. Individuals who become a member of new subcultures will, like the soldiers, find themselves removed from their normal social environment and many of their social and moral restraints. They will be submerged into the moral and social codes of the sub culture, which will differ from the more mainstream morals and social codes. However it is clear that not all people become addicts because of a change of setting, or because of a traumatic experience.

"Availability is such as obvious determinant of drug taking that it is often overlooked." (Gossip, M. 2007:33) It could be assumed that the more available an item is, the more it will be used. Rationale addiction theory explains how availability and price affects addiction. It adds another dimension to the understanding of addiction. "According to the theory, past prices will affect present consumption... The theory also predicts that the addict is forward looking and that they will adjust consumption in advance, when anticipating future price changes. If the agent expects that prices will go up in the future, they are expected to start reducing consumption immediately, and if a reduction is anticipated, they are expected to increase consumption. (Skog, O. et al, 2006:1444) This theory shows that addicts do in fact keep their free will, and their addiction is a rationale one, which is based upon the availability of drugs, and at a price which suits their lifestyles. This will not apply to everyone however as those who have the money to support an addiction no matter the cost will not need to be as forward thinking.

It is clear that their cannot be one universal understanding of addiction. The disease model explains how the body reacts and adapts to addiction, but does not explain the start of addiction or why it begins. The social model explains why addictions may develop, and how they are not so much a disease, but a coping mechanism for those trying to escape the world they live in. The rational choice theory shows that addiction does not extinguish free will, but does not account for those who can support an addiction all year round. It is clear "[t]he concept of addiction is unhelpful: it suggests a dependency with grave consequences for the individual and society, Not all drug users develop dependency...the term 'problem drug user' is therefore increasingly favoured." (Scott, J. 2009:193-194) However this in itself causes an issue, what is a problem to one person may not be to another. It can be argued that there should not be a universal understanding of addiction, as each case of addiction will always, even if only slightly, be unique.

Bibliography

Alexander, B. (N.D), A Historical Analysis of Addiction,
<http://www.nad.fi/pdf/44/Bruce%20K.%20Alexander.pdf> Date accessed 01/01/2010

Boyd, J. (1999), Addiction Faith Without Works, The Centre for Bioethics and Human Dignity,
<http://www.defeataddictions.org/files/Addiction_Faith_Without_Works.pdf> date accessed
21/12/2009

Deans, D. (1997), Drug Addiction, California State University,
<http://www.csun.edu/~vcpsy00h/students/drugs.htm> Date accessed 30/12/2009

Eysenck, H. (1997), Addiction, Personality and Motivation, Human Psychopharmacology, Vol.
12:79-87, <http://www3.interscience.wiley.com/cgi-bin/fulltext/30001300/PDFSTART>

Gori, G. (1996), Failings of the Disease Model of Addiction, Human Psychopharmacology, Vol.
11: 33-38,
<http://www.fungerendeliv.no/Artikler/pdf/failings%20of%20the%20disease%20model.pdf> date
accessed 24/12/2009

Gossop, M. (2007), Living with Drugs, (6th edn), Hampshire, Ashgate Publishing Limited

Heyman, G. (2009), Resolving The Contradictions Of Addiction,
<http://www.defeataddictions.org/files/RESOLVING_THE_CONTRADICTIONS_OF_ADDICTION.
pdf> date accessed 22/12/2009

Hyman, S. & Malenka, R. (2001), Addiction and the Brain: The Neurobiology of Compulsion and
its Persistence, Nature Reviews, Vol. 2: 695- 703,
<http://www.sacklerinstitute.org/cornell/summer_institute/2005/papers/hyman2001.pdf> date
accessed 21/12/2009

Kerr, J. (1996), Two Myths of Addiction: The Addictive Personality and the Issue of Free Choice,
Human Psychopharmacology, Vol 11:9-13,
<http://www3.interscience.wiley.com/cgi-bin/fulltext/21069/PDFSTART>

5

Lavine, H. (1978), The Discovery Of Addiction Changing Conceptions Of Habitual Drunkenness In America, <u>Journal of Studies on Alcohol</u>, Vol. 15:493-506, <http://www.defeataddictions.org/files/THE_DISCOVERY_OF_ADDICTION.pdf> date accessed 22/12/2009

Lende, D & Smith, E. (2001), Evolution meets biopsyosociality: an analysis of addictive behaviour, <u>Addiction</u>, Vol 97, (4): 447-458, <http://www3.interscience.wiley.com/cgi-bin/fulltext/118957989/PDFSTART>

Scott, J. & Marshall, G. (2009), <u>Oxford Dictionary Of Sociology</u>, (3rd edn revisited) Oxford, Oxford University Press

Skog, O. & Melberg, H. (2006), Becker's rational addiction theory: an empirical test with price elasticities for distilled spirits in Denmark 1911–31, <u>Addiction</u>, Vol 101(10):1444–1450, <http://www3.interscience.wiley.com/cgi-bin/fulltext/118730527/PDFSTART>

Val, P. (2009), Addiction - and rational choice theory, <u>International Journal of Consumer Studies</u>, Blackwell Publishing LTD, <http://www3.interscience.wiley.com/cgi-bin/fulltext/122683837/PDFSTART>

'questionable' in its relevance to meaningful democratic citizenship; the listing of prime ministers and naming of famous Canadians was cited among other "arcane historical and political facts" (p. 18). Although respecting the potential problems associated with these perceived areas of ignorance in the Canadian population, Sears and Hyslop-Margison dismiss this as a crisis of citizenship stating that this knowledge is "not particularly essential to good citizenship" (p. 18).

Turning to the crisis of alienation, the authors refer to a conclusion of alienation from the socio-political apparatus that has been drawn, primarily, from steadily declining voter participation rates, especially among younger voters. Sears and Hyslop-Margison in essence endeavor to sever the idea of political alienation from that of civic alienation. Pointing to research that suggests contemporary youth are no more cynical than their parents, but rather less allegiant to partisan politics, concluding that today's youth are merely alienated from a "political system closed to meaningful consultation and participation" (Buckingham, 1999, as cited on p. 18). They proceed to illustrate that this does not translate into across-the-board civic disengagement, but does perhaps reflect the significant voter decline. In fact, the authors turn to Gautier (2002) to demonstrate that youth are turning to a form of participatory democracy; they are engaging in social movements such as environmentalism, and that this form of civic engagement is increasing. Thus, our youth have merely shifted their participation away from the purely political process to a more "grass roots" form of engagement.

Finally, in respect to the crisis of agnosticism, Sears and Hyslop-Margison argue that we cannot conclude, from such incidents as "ethically motivated attacks on foreign residents in Canada, Europe, and the United States" a "serious deficit of democratic values" (p. 20). Arguing that the situation is not this simple, the authors defer to a host of studies that have identified youth as "positive" towards an expanse of democratic values. In fact, they point to the willingness of youth to limit rights such as freedom of speech for groups promoting racism. Recognizing that some may see this denial of access as a low level commitment to fundamental democratic values, Sears and Hyslop-Margison respond by saying that it does demonstrate that young people are "genuinely concerned with ethno-cultural diversity" (p. 20). They end simply with a statement that the crisis of agnosticism is complex.

In their general conclusion to the article authors Alan Sears and Emery Hyslop-Margison reassert that there is a need to move from cult mentality (sweeping and unfounded generalizations, slogans and rhetoric) to a critical and reliable analysis of citizenship education reform. The problems arise when we begin to understand the *ipso facto* landscape of citizenship they have created in illustrating this point. In attempting to make a case for a careful, nuanced, and holistic analysis of citizenship education, the authors have actually proven the ease with which academic discourse can gloss over the very complexities they endeavored to highlight.

In their response to the crisis of ignorance, the authors do not consider the degree to which our youth understand, or do not understand, contemporary socio-political issues. I would assert that there is indeed a crisis of ignorance in this area. Political and historical facts are crucial "nuts and bolts" in the forming of complex understandings of contemporary issues. Further, there is much evidence to support the idea that the knowledge young people do have is disconnected from meaningful contexts. They are without a fundamental foundation of liberal education which allows a synchronization of knowledge to arrive at authentic understandings of complex situations. (see, for example, Hyslop-Margison, 2005). This becomes crucial when we turn to their arguments regarding the crisis of alienation. How might today's youth make a serious and meaningful impact by way of various social movements, such as environmentalism as the authors allude to, if they are without a genuine understanding of the fundamental nature at the heart of the problem? Further, how effective can any form of protest be without any meaningful connection to, or understanding of, the apparatus of governance which, ultimately, will need to be involved in substantial change to something like the environment which is essentially political? (see, for instance, Orr., 2004) To use the words of Sears and Hyslop-Margison there must be a balance with "the dispositional requirements of meaningful political engagement" and not simply a passing awareness of its function (p. 16). In effect, alienated from a political system, regardless of its nature or effectiveness, these youth are merely preaching to the converted- a general populace who, if also alienated from the political structure, are powerless to evoke any form of substantial change on a systemic level. Additionally, the authors leave us with a sense of the problem being exclusively that of the political structure and quote Osborne (2000) who in effect states that the problem rests with the political system and that the change is needed there and cannot be effected through better citizenship education.

This seems rather incongruous with fundamental concept of citizenship education. Is the idea not to change societal institutions, such as those which form 'government', by way of a more effective citizenry? Is change not effected by humans and are all humans not first and foremost citizens?

Within the crisis of agnosticism authors Sears and Hyslop-Margison again reduce the issue to a form of black and white in many respects. In response to a claim that our youth lack commitment to democratic virtues the authors provide research tantamount to a mere enumeration of democratic values knowledge among the youth population. The essential aspect they neglect is that identification of, or even an abstract understanding of democratic values does not equate to a "genuine" embodiment of the democratic spirit. I would refer to a quote provided by the authors elsewhere in the article which states that "don't teach us about the forms of democracy, we know all about the forms of democracy, we need to learn the spirit of democracy" (Herman, 1996, as quoted on p. 17). In fact, one might defer here to the work of these authors throughout their academic careers which have essentially established that our schools are teaching decontextualized democratic values (see, for example, Sears and Hughes, 1996; Hyslop-Margison and Graham, 2001; Hyslop-Margison, 2005). Thus, it should come as no surprise that our youth can reiterate them on survey upon survey. Being asked a question on a survey best resembles a test question whereby students are asked to reiterate information. Of course, they will supply an answer that is accepting and open towards immigrants, for instance, if that is what they have memorized, but this in no way equates to an evaluation of their "attitudes" which are truly manifest. Although I agree that the participants presenting a conflict in their support or free speech versus its actual application does not equate to a lack of commitment, I would suggest that it establishes their lack of internalization, and does not translate to a "genuine concern" as the authors would suggest.

In the end, the authors do not dismiss concern with the discourse of agnosticism, but they have given support to the idea that our youth are genuinely concerned with democratic values beyond that which we give them credit. The problem is that this assumption is based on information that simply reflects their awareness of the values and not their embodiment of such.

Although I give credit to the authors for hinting towards this dilemma throughout the article, I am disappointed that it did not figure into the discussion on agnosticism more deliberately. This is the very seat of the crisis in democratic citizenship.

Alan Sears and Emery Hyslop-Margison do succeed in forwarding a solid case for the need to take a much more nuanced, careful, and holistic look at democratic citizenship education reform. However, there is a sense of calm and "all-right-ness" emanating from this work that I would suggest is gravely dangerous. In over-simplifying the discourse of crises the authors have dismissed with the urgency rather than making it more exacting. Although, much of the "discourse of crisis" surrounding democratic citizenship and citizenship education may be off the mark, as they have established in many instances, this should not translate to an underestimation of the degree of urgency surrounding the problematics of genuine democratic engagement and civic virtue in contemporary youth. We do need to dispense with the cult mentality and its slogans and rhetoric, but in doing so we cannot afford to diminish the sense of crisis.

Perhaps the events of September 13, 2006 at Dawson College in Montreal where a young man opened fire on innocent, random students, gives substance to this disconnect between being theoretically aware of versus truly embodying human virtue. The various desirable dispositions of democratic citizenship, such as acceptance of diversity, can only truly manifest when experienced in relations to others. This connection between humans, as a virtue building exercise, is crucial. Contemporary democracy and capitalist economies have greatly diminished this by encouraging individual isolation and as a result young Canadians may "know" democratic virtues, but do not embody them in their very essence. It is this absence of *praxis* that should concern us with great urgency; concern us with a sense of crisis.

References

Hyslop-Margison, E. J. (2005). *Liberalizing vocational study: Democratic approaches to career education.* Lanham, MD: University Press of America.

Hyslop-Margison, E. J., & Graham, B. (2001). Principles for democratic learning in career education. *Canadian Journal of Education, 26*(3).

Orr, D. W. (2004). *Earth in mind: On education, environment, and the human prospect.* Washington, DC: Island Press.

Pinsky, R. (2002). *Democracy, culture and the voice of poetry.* Princeton, NJ: Princeton University Press.

Sears, A. M., & Hughes, A. S. (1996). Citizenship education and current educational reform. *Canadian Journal of Education, 21*(2).

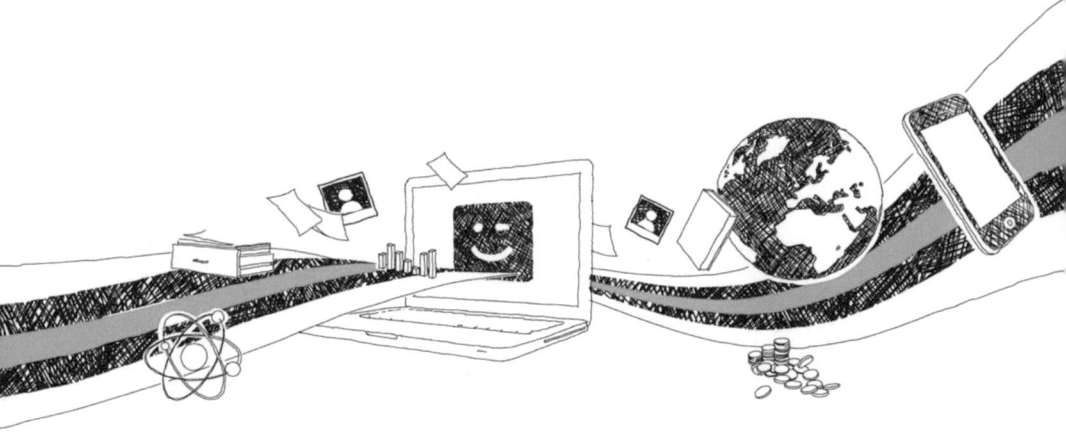
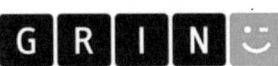